Sodium Control for Seniors

A Comprehensive Guide to Managing Salt for Better Health and Longevity, With a Sample 7-Day Meal Plan and Recipes copyright © 2025 Mary Golanna

All rights reserved No part of this book may be reproduced, or stored in a retrieval system, or transmitted in any form or by any means, electronic, mechanical, photocopying, recording, or otherwise, without express written permission of the publisher.

Disclaimer

By reading this disclaimer, you are accepting the terms of the disclaimer in full. If you disagree with this disclaimer, please do not read the guide.

All of the content within this guide is provided for informational and educational purposes only, and should not be accepted as independent medical or other professional advice. The author is not a doctor, physician, nurse, mental health provider, or registered nutritionist/dietician. Therefore, using and reading this guide does not establish any form of a physician-patient relationship.

Always consult with a physician or another qualified health provider with any issues or questions you might have regarding any sort of medical condition. Do not ever disregard any qualified professional medical advice or delay seeking that advice because of anything you have read in this guide. The information in this guide is not intended to be any sort of medical advice and should not be used in lieu of any medical advice by a licensed and qualified medical professional.

The information in this guide has been compiled from a variety of known sources. However, the author cannot attest to or guarantee the accuracy of each source and thus should not be held liable for any errors or omissions.

You acknowledge that the publisher of this guide will not be held liable for any loss or damage of any kind incurred as a result of this guide or the reliance on any information provided within this guide. You acknowledge and agree that you assume all risk and responsibility for any action you undertake in response to the information in this guide.

Using this guide does not guarantee any particular result (e.g., weight loss or a cure). By reading this guide, you acknowledge that there are no guarantees to any specific outcome or results you can expect.

All product names, diet plans, or names used in this guide are for identification purposes only and are the property of their respective owners. The use of these names does not imply endorsement. All other trademarks cited herein are the property of their respective owners.

Where applicable, this guide is not intended to be a substitute for the original work of this diet plan and is, at most, a supplement to the original work for this diet plan and never a direct substitute. This guide is a personal expression of the facts of that diet plan.

Where applicable, persons shown in the cover images are stock photography models and the publisher has obtained the rights to use the images through license agreements with third-party stock image companies.

Table of Contents

Introduction	8
The Science of Sodium: What You Need to Know	10
How Sodium Affects Blood Pressure	10
Sodium and Heart, Kidney, and Bone Health	11
Recommended Daily Sodium Intake for Seniors	12
Signs of Too Much Sodium	15
Recognizing Symptoms of Sodium Overload	15
The Impact of Sodium on Chronic Conditions	16
Practical Tips for Managing Sodium	18
Low Sodium vs. No Sodium - What's Right for You?	19
What's the Difference Between Low Sodium and No Sodium?	19
The Importance of Finding Balance	20
How to Determine the Best Option for You	20
Practical Tips for Getting the Balance Right	21
How to Reduce Sodium in Your Diet	23
Easy Swaps for High-Sodium Foods	23
The Best Salt Substitutes for Seniors	25
Tips for Maintaining Flavor	26
Reading Labels Like a Pro	27
Decoding Nutrition Facts	27
Hidden Sources of Sodium in Everyday Foods	28
Tips for Making Smart Choices	29
Cooking Low-Sodium Meals at Home	31
Essential Ingredients for Sodium Control	31
Tips for Enhancing Flavor Without Salt	33
Dining Out Without Worry	36
How to Communicate Your Needs	38
7-Day Low-Sodium Meal Plan for Seniors	41

Day 1	41
Day 2	42
Day 3	42
Day 4	42
Day 5	43
Day 6	43
Day 7	44
Final Tips for Success	44
Quick and Easy Low-Sodium Recipes	**45**
Lentil and Spinach Soup	46
Creamy Avocado and Cucumber Salad	47
Tomato Basil Soup	48
Rainbow Quinoa Salad	49
Vegetable Barley Soup	50
Lemon Herb Chicken	51
Grilled Salmon with Dill Sauce	53
Stuffed Bell Peppers	54
Zucchini Noodles with Garlic Shrimp	56
Vegetarian Stir-Fry	57
Turkey and Avocado Wrap	58
Rosemary Pork Chops	59
Vegetable and Chickpea Curry	60
Baked Cod with Lemon and Garlic	61
Beef and Vegetable Skewers	62
Fresh Berry Yogurt Parfait	63
Baked Apples with Cinnamon	64
Chia Seed Pudding	65
Banana Ice Cream	66
Dark Chocolate-Dipped Strawberries	67
Tracking Your Sodium Intake	**68**
Journals, Apps, and Tools for Seniors	68

Staying Consistent	70
Dealing with Cravings and Setbacks	71
Tips for Managing Salt Cravings	72
Staying Motivated	74
When to Consult a Doctor or Dietitian	**75**
Medical Conditions	75
Plateaus or Challenges	76
Custom Plans	78
Recognizing When You Need Help	79
Conclusion	**84**
FAQs	**87**
References and Helpful Links	**90**

Introduction

Sodium often flies under the radar when considering key nutrients for overall health. Most of us think of it as the sprinkle of salt that enhances the flavor of our favorite dishes. But sodium plays a much larger role than simply seasoning food—especially as we age. It's a vital electrolyte that supports critical bodily functions, from maintaining fluid balance to keeping our muscles and nerves working properly.

However, the way our bodies process sodium can change over time. Aging impacts kidney function, making it harder to regulate sodium levels efficiently. This shift means seniors face greater challenges in managing sodium intake, and striking the right balance becomes essential. Low levels can lead to issues like fatigue and muscle weakness, while too much sodium can contribute to high blood pressure, heart strain, and an increased risk of chronic disease.

Despite sodium's importance, plenty of myths surround it, particularly for older adults. Some believe seniors must entirely cut salt out of their diets, while others assume their lifelong habits need no adjustment at all. These misconceptions can lead to confusion, causing seniors to either restrict sodium unnecessarily or unknowingly face health risks from overindulgence.

In this guide, we will talk about the following:

- The Science of Sodium: What You Need to Know
- Signs of Too Much Sodium
- Low Sodium vs. No Sodium: What's Right for You?
- How to Reduce Sodium in Your Diet
- Cooking Low-Sodium Meals at Home
- Dining Out Without Worry
- 7-Day Low-Sodium Meal Plan for Seniors and Quick and Easy Low-Sodium Recipes
- Tracking Your Sodium Intake
- Dealing with Cravings and Setbacks
- When to Consult a Doctor or Dietitian

Keep reading to learn more about how sodium impacts the aging body and what seniors can do to maintain healthy levels for a happier, healthier life. By understanding the science behind sodium and its effects on our bodies, we can make informed decisions about our diets and take control of our health as we age.

The Science of Sodium: What You Need to Know

Sodium is one of the body's key electrolytes—minerals that carry an electric charge to help with essential body functions. It interacts with potassium to regulate fluid balance, ensuring water is distributed properly across cells and tissues. It also helps send nerve signals and keeps muscles, including the heart, working smoothly.

The body carefully manages sodium levels through the kidneys, which adjusts how much sodium is retained or excreted. However, as people age, kidney function may decline, impacting the ability to maintain this balance. This means seniors may have a greater sensitivity to sodium, making moderation even more important.

How Sodium Affects Blood Pressure

Sodium has a direct relationship with blood pressure. When you consume too much sodium, the body holds onto extra water to dilute it. This increases the volume of blood, leading to higher blood pressure. For seniors, high blood pressure—or hypertension—poses a significant risk, as it can lead to heart disease, stroke, or other complications.

On the flip side, not getting enough sodium can also be problematic. Low sodium levels in the body, known as hyponatremia, can occur, particularly if medications or health conditions affect sodium processing. Symptoms can include fatigue, confusion, and even more serious issues like falls, which are especially concerning for older adults. That's why finding the right sodium balance is key.

Sodium and Heart, Kidney, and Bone Health

Beyond blood pressure, sodium influences other critical areas of health.

- *Heart Health*: High sodium intake can strain the cardiovascular system, contributing to conditions like heart failure, where the heart struggles to pump blood effectively. For seniors, who are already at higher risk for heart problems, managing sodium is a crucial part of keeping the heart healthy.
- *Kidney Health*: Kidneys are responsible for filtering sodium out of the bloodstream. If they have to process too much, it can overwork them, potentially worsening conditions like chronic kidney disease (CKD), which is common in seniors. On the other hand, inadequate sodium can also impact kidney function, highlighting the need for balance.

- ***Bone Health***: A lesser-known impact of high sodium intake is its effect on bones. Excess sodium can lead to calcium loss through urine. Over time, this can weaken bones and increase the risk of osteoporosis, a condition many seniors are already prone to. Keeping sodium within recommended levels can help protect bone density.

It's clear that sodium plays a significant role in multiple aspects of health, and finding the right balance is essential for seniors to maintain overall well-being.

Recommended Daily Sodium Intake for Seniors

The recommended daily sodium intake for seniors generally falls around 1,500 to 2,300 milligrams, depending on individual health needs. For context, one teaspoon of salt contains about 2,300 milligrams of sodium.

Seniors with conditions like high blood pressure, heart disease, or kidney problems should aim for the lower end of the range. Those who are generally healthy can stick to the higher end, but it's still wise to avoid excess.

Here are some practical tips for managing sodium intake effectively:

- ***Read food labels***: Processed and packaged foods often contain hidden sources of sodium that can add up quickly. Take the time to check nutrition labels for the sodium content and aim for options with lower sodium per serving. Be especially cautious with canned soups, frozen meals, and snack foods, which are known to be high-sodium culprits.

- ***Cook fresh meals***: Preparing your meals with fresh ingredients like fruits, vegetables, whole grains, and lean proteins not only keeps sodium levels low but also ensures you're eating more nutrient-dense, wholesome food. Fresh ingredients naturally contain minimal sodium, and cooking at home gives you full control over how much salt is added (if any).
- ***Use herbs and spices***: Instead of relying on salt to enhance the flavor of your food, try experimenting with a variety of herbs, spices, and other natural seasonings. Garlic, pepper, parsley, basil, rosemary, cumin, and turmeric are just a few flavorful options that can elevate your meals without adding unnecessary sodium. You might also try using citrus like lemon or lime juice for a zesty kick.
- ***Be mindful of condiments***: Many condiments, such as soy sauce, ketchup, salad dressings, and barbecue sauces, are surprisingly high in sodium. Use these sparingly or look for low-sodium or reduced-sodium alternatives. You can also try making your own condiments at home, which allows you to customize the flavor while controlling the sodium content.

By understanding the science behind sodium and its effects on the body, seniors can make informed dietary decisions. Striking the right balance ensures better blood pressure control, heart and kidney health, and stronger bones—all key to living a healthier, more vibrant life.

Signs of Too Much Sodium

When someone consumes too much sodium, the body reacts in different ways. One of the earliest signs is fluid retention, which may cause bloating, swelling in the hands and feet, or puffiness around the face. This happens because sodium causes the body to retain extra water to balance itself out.

Another common sign is increased thirst. A high-sodium meal can leave you feeling extra thirsty as the body tries to rehydrate and dilute the sodium levels in your blood. Related to this is frequent urination, as the kidneys work to flush the excess sodium.

Over time, unchecked sodium intake can lead to more severe signs like elevated blood pressure, persistent headaches, or shortness of breath, which signal a strain on the cardiovascular system.

Recognizing Symptoms of Sodium Overload

The symptoms of sodium overload may not always be easy to spot, but paying attention to your body's signals can make a big difference. For seniors, it's particularly important to watch for recurring fatigue or confusion. These symptoms can sometimes indicate an imbalance caused by sodium levels being too high.

Swelling in the lower extremities, like ankles and feet, can develop when the body retains too much fluid. High sodium intake can also worsen existing symptoms for those with preexisting conditions like high blood pressure or heart disease.

It's crucial to recognize symptoms early, as sodium overload can escalate into more severe complications, such as hospitalization for heart failure or difficulties managing other chronic conditions.

The Impact of Sodium on Chronic Conditions

Excessive sodium doesn't just cause short-term discomfort — it can have serious long-term consequences, especially for seniors with chronic health conditions.

- ***Heart Disease***: High sodium levels increase blood pressure, which puts added strain on the heart and blood vessels. Over time, this added pressure can damage the cardiovascular system, leading to an increased risk of heart disease, strokes, or heart failure. These conditions tend to become more common with age, making it especially important for seniors to monitor their sodium intake to protect their heart health and overall circulation.

- *Kidney Disease*: The kidneys play a vital role in filtering and eliminating excess sodium from the body, maintaining a healthy balance. For seniors with chronic kidney disease (CKD), consuming too much sodium can overload the kidneys, worsening their function and accelerating the progression of the disease. This can also lead to fluid retention and elevated blood pressure, further complicating health issues.
- *Osteoporosis*: A less obvious but significant impact of high sodium is its effect on bone health. When sodium levels in the body are too high, it can cause increased calcium excretion through urine. Over time, this gradual calcium loss can weaken bones, decreasing bone density and raising the risk of fractures. For aging individuals, maintaining bone health is critical to preserving mobility and preventing injuries.

Seniors with multiple chronic conditions may experience compounded effects when sodium intake isn't managed. For example, high sodium could worsen both kidney disease and high blood pressure at the same time, making overall disease management even harder.

Practical Tips for Managing Sodium

Reducing sodium intake is one of the most effective ways to avoid these problems. Here are some simple but effective tips to keep sodium levels in check:

- *Limit processed foods*: Prepackaged foods like canned soups, frozen meals, and snacks are often packed with sodium. Choose fresh, whole foods whenever possible.
- *Check labels*: Foods labeled as "low-sodium" or "sodium-free" can help reduce unexpected sodium. Always read the nutrition information.
- *Prepare meals at home*: Cooking meals from scratch gives you full control over sodium content. Use herbs and spices to add flavor instead of salt.
- *Watch your condiments*: Soy sauce, ketchup, salad dressings, and other condiments can be surprisingly high in sodium. Use these sparingly or choose low-sodium versions.
- *Stay hydrated*: Drinking enough water helps your body balance sodium levels and flush any excess.

By recognizing the signs of sodium overload, understanding how it affects chronic conditions, and following simple management techniques, seniors can better protect their health. Moderation and balance are the keys to keeping sodium in check and ensuring a healthier, more comfortable life.

Low Sodium vs. No Sodium - What's Right for You?

When it comes to managing sodium intake, the idea of cutting back can feel overwhelming. Do you need to completely eliminate sodium, or would simply reducing it be enough? Finding the balance between low sodium and no sodium is key, especially for seniors whose nutritional needs change with age. Understanding these options and tailoring them to your health can help you make informed choices.

What's the Difference Between Low Sodium and No Sodium?

A low-sodium diet minimizes sodium intake but doesn't eliminate it altogether. This approach typically aims for about 1,500–2,300 milligrams of sodium per day, which aligns with recommendations for those managing conditions like high blood pressure, kidney disease, or heart issues. Lowering sodium helps reduce water retention, manage blood pressure, and support overall cardiovascular health.

A no-sodium diet, on the other hand, involves cutting out as much sodium as possible. While this might seem like the ultimate solution, it can be challenging to follow and, in some cases, unnecessary. Sodium is an essential mineral that the body needs to maintain fluid balance, send nerve signals, and assist muscle function. Removing it completely can lead to problems like muscle cramps, confusion, or fatigue — especially for seniors who may already have sensitive dietary needs.

The Importance of Finding Balance

The "right" amount of sodium isn't the same for everyone. It depends on your individual health conditions and requirements. For example, if you have hypertension, your doctor might recommend a low-sodium diet to help control your blood pressure. However, cutting sodium entirely isn't typically necessary. The goal is moderation, not elimination.

Similarly, people taking diuretic medications or with specific health conditions may need slightly more sodium to avoid issues like hyponatremia, a condition where sodium levels drop too low. This is why it's so important to approach sodium intake as a balance, not a one-size-fits-all rule.

How to Determine the Best Option for You

Determining your ideal sodium intake starts with a conversation with your healthcare provider. They can help assess your overall health, activity level, and any underlying conditions. Based on this, they will recommend a sodium target tailored to your needs.

If a low-sodium diet is recommended, aim to stick to the target range without restricting sodium completely. Learn to read food labels, as packaged foods often contain hidden sodium even when they don't taste overly salty. Look for items labeled as "low sodium" and aim for fresh, unprocessed foods where possible.

For those who may temporarily need an extremely low-sodium or no-sodium diet, such as during treatment for specific medical issues, your doctor or dietitian can guide you on how to maintain proper hydration and nutrient balance.

Practical Tips for Getting the Balance Right

Making dietary changes might seem daunting, but it doesn't have to be. Here are some practical ideas for implementing a low-sodium lifestyle while keeping your meals enjoyable and varied:

- *Cook fresh meals*: Start with whole foods like vegetables, fruits, lean meats, or fish. These naturally contain little to no sodium and are packed with essential nutrients.
- *Use alternative seasoning*: Skip the salt shaker and try herbs, spices, lemon, or vinegar to enhance flavors.

Garlic, onion powder, and smoked paprika can make a meal flavorful without added sodium.
- ***Limit processed foods***: Items like canned soups, frozen dinners, and deli meats are high in sodium. Look for reduced-sodium options or prepare your own versions at home.
- ***Wash off canned items***: Washing canned vegetables and beans under cold water can reduce their sodium content by up to 40%.
- ***Be mindful of "hidden" sodium***: Many condiments and sauces, like soy sauce, ketchup, or salad dressings, pack a surprising sodium punch. Use them sparingly or make your own at home.

Low sodium versus no sodium isn't a battle where one option wins. It's about understanding what's best for your health and making sustainable changes that take your body's needs into account. For most seniors, low-sodium diets provide the right balance — reducing health risks while still allowing the body to get the sodium it needs to function properly.

With planning and smart choices, reducing sodium doesn't mean sacrificing flavor or convenience. It means taking control of your diet to support your health and lead a vibrant, active life at any age. Always consult with a healthcare provider before making significant dietary changes to ensure you're on the best path for your individual needs.

How to Reduce Sodium in Your Diet

Cutting back on sodium doesn't mean sacrificing taste or enjoying meals less. For seniors, reducing sodium is a crucial part of maintaining health, especially in managing blood pressure, heart issues, and kidney health. Luckily, making simple changes in your diet can significantly lower sodium intake while keeping meals flavorful and satisfying.

Easy Swaps for High-Sodium Foods

Many foods we eat every day contain hidden sodium. Processed and packaged items tend to be sneaky culprits. Here are some easy swaps to reduce sodium while still enjoying delicious meals:

- *Bread and Baked Goods*: High sodium levels can lurk in bread and baked goods. Opt for whole-grain or low-sodium bread options. You can also bake your own bread at home to control how much salt goes in.
- *Canned and Packaged Soups*: Many soups are high in sodium. Swap them for homemade versions made with

fresh ingredients and low-sodium broth. If you use canned soups, look for reduced-sodium options and add a splash of fresh lemon or your favorite herbs for extra flavor.

- *Processed Meats*: Deli meats, bacon, sausages, and hot dogs are packed with sodium. Try fresh alternatives like roasted chicken or turkey breast. You can also season and roast lean cuts of meat at home to replace processed options.
- *Cheese*: Many cheeses, especially processed ones, are sodium-heavy. Swap for lower-sodium versions like mozzarella or Swiss cheese, or reduce portion sizes while enhancing flavors with other foods like fresh veggies.
- *Salty Snacks*: Instead of potato chips or pretzels, try air-popped popcorn seasoned with herbs, unsalted nuts, or veggie sticks with hummus for a satisfying crunch.
- *Condiments*: Soy sauce, ketchup, salad dressings, and barbecue sauces often add lots of sodium. Look for low-sodium versions or make your own condiments at home using simple ingredients.

Overall, being mindful of hidden sodium sources and making small changes in our daily food choices can help reduce our sodium intake without sacrificing flavor.

The Best Salt Substitutes for Seniors

Reducing sodium doesn't mean your meals have to be bland. Many salt substitutes and natural flavor boosters can make food just as enjoyable while keeping sodium in check. Here are some great options for seniors:

- *Herbs and Spices*: Fresh or dried herbs like basil, rosemary, thyme, and oregano are fantastic for boosting flavor. Spices like cumin, paprika, and turmeric add depth and complexity to dishes without relying on salt.
- *Citrus Zest and Juice*: A squeeze of lemon, lime, or orange juice can brighten up a meal. Grated citrus zest can also pack a powerful punch of flavor, perfect for salads, roasted veggies, or fish.
- *Vinegar*: Balsamic, apple cider, or red wine vinegar can bring tangy depth to dishes. Use them in marinades, salad dressings, or for drizzling over roasted vegetables.
- *Garlic and Onion*: Fresh garlic and onion—or their powdered forms without added salt—can add a rich, savory taste to just about any dish.
- *Smoked Paprika or Ground Mustard*: Both ingredients provide bold, smoky, or tangy flavors, making them perfect substitutes for seasoning meats, veggies, or even popcorn.

- *Umami Builds*: Mushrooms, nutritional yeast, tomato paste, or unsalted soy sauce bring an umami-packed richness to your meals. Use them generously to add that "fifth flavor" sensation.

These salt substitutes are just some of the many options seniors can use to season their food without relying on sodium. Experiment with different combinations and find what works best for your taste buds.

Tips for Maintaining Flavor

Reducing sodium doesn't mean the food should taste bland. Focus on layering flavors instead of relying on salt. Start with fresh, high-quality ingredients that have their own natural flavors. Slowly introduce substitutes like herbs, citrus, or spices, and taste as you go. Cooking techniques like roasting or grilling can also enhance the natural sweetness and depth of foods, making dishes taste even better.

Finally, remember that it's all about balance. Gradually reduce sodium intake over time, and your taste buds will adjust. With these easy swaps and flavorful substitutes, seniors can enjoy satisfying, health-conscious meals that nourish both the body and the soul.

Reading Labels Like a Pro

Taking control of sodium intake starts with knowing what's in your food. Nutrition labels hold the key, but decoding them can feel like sorting through a puzzle. With a little knowledge, you can read labels like a pro and spot hidden sources of sodium in everyday foods.

Decoding Nutrition Facts

The Nutrition Facts label on packaged foods is your best tool for managing sodium consumption. Here's how to break it down step by step:

- ***Serving Size***: Always check the serving size first. The sodium amount listed applies to one serving, not the entire package. If you eat double the serving size, you're also doubling the sodium intake.
- ***Sodium Content***: Sodium is listed in milligrams (mg). A good general rule is to aim for foods with 140 mg or less per serving, which is considered low sodium. Be cautious with foods that have 20% or more of the daily value (DV) for sodium in a single serving, as these are high in sodium.

- *% Daily Value (%DV)*: The percentage next to sodium shows how much it contributes to your recommended daily intake, based on a 2,300 mg daily limit. For many seniors, doctors may recommend staying closer to 1,500 mg per day, so adjust accordingly.
- *Ingredient List*: Sodium isn't just listed as "salt." Look for terms like monosodium glutamate (MSG), sodium bicarbonate, or sodium nitrate in the ingredient list. These are all forms of sodium that add to your intake.

Overall, the key is to pay attention to serving sizes and %DV and choose foods lower in sodium. This can help you make more informed choices about what you eat and how it affects your health.

Hidden Sources of Sodium in Everyday Foods

Sodium isn't always obvious. Many foods you wouldn't think of as salty could have significant amounts of hidden sodium. Here are some common sources to watch for:

- *Bread and Baked Goods*: A single slice of bread can contain 100-200 mg of sodium. Some "healthier" options like whole-grain bread can still pack a lot of salt.
- *Canned Vegetables and Soups*: Even vegetables can come loaded with sodium to preserve freshness. Soups

are one of the worst offenders, with some cans containing over 700 mg per serving.
- *Frozen Meals*: Convenience comes at a cost. Many frozen meals, even "diet" or "healthy" ones, can have over half the recommended daily sodium intake in a single serving.
- *Sauces and Condiments*: Soy sauce, ketchup, barbecue sauce, and salad dressings are sneaky sources. Just one tablespoon can pack as much as 200-300 mg of sodium.
- *Cheese and Dairy*: Cheese, especially processed varieties like American or parmesan, can contain significant sodium. Always check the label, even for products marketed as lower fat.
- *Snacks*: Chips, crackers, and even "healthy" snacks like veggie chips can have hidden sodium. Even sweet treats like cookies can surprise you with added salt.

Overall, it's important to check labels and be mindful of sodium content in all foods. Even seemingly innocuous items like bread or soup can add up quickly throughout the day. Opting for homemade meals and using herbs and spices instead of salt can help reduce your overall intake.

Tips for Making Smart Choices

Now that you know where hidden sources of sodium can be found, here are some tips for making smarter choices:

- ***Opt for Fresh Foods***: They're your best options for keeping sodium under control.
- ***Choose Lower-Sodium Options***: Many brands now offer reduced-sodium or no-salt-added versions of common items like canned vegetables, soups, and condiments. Make these your go-to choices.
- ***Beware of "Hidden" Sodium Claims***: Just because a product claims to be "low-fat" or "organic" doesn't mean it's low in sodium. Always check the label to be sure.
- ***Wash Off Canned Items***: Washing canned beans or vegetables thoroughly under cold water can reduce their sodium content by as much as 40%.
- ***Flavor Without Salt***: Use herbs, spices, and citrus to flavor your food instead of relying on salty sauces or seasonings.

Learning to read food labels and spot hidden sodium helps you make better decisions and reduce intake without giving up the flavors you love. Over time, these small changes can make a big impact on your health, especially for seniors aiming to manage blood pressure and improve heart and kidney health. With practice, you can confidently read labels like a pro and take control of your diet.

Cooking Low-Sodium Meals at Home

Preparing meals at home gives you full control over what goes into your food, and that's one of the best ways to reduce sodium in your diet. For seniors, this becomes even more important as managing sodium can help protect the heart, kidneys, and overall health. By choosing the right ingredients and learning to enhance flavor in creative ways, you can make delicious, low-sodium meals that the whole family will enjoy.

Essential Ingredients for Sodium Control

When cooking at home, building your pantry and fridge with the right ingredients is step one. These items will help you create flavorful, low-sodium dishes without compromising on taste.

- *Fresh or Frozen Vegetables*: Go for fresh or frozen vegetables without added sauces or seasonings. They naturally contain little to no sodium and pack plenty of flavor and nutrients. Look for options like spinach,

broccoli, carrots, and peppers to keep meal prep interesting.
- **Whole Grains**: Choose unprocessed whole grains like brown rice, quinoa, and oats. These have no added sodium and serve as a hearty, filling base for any meal.
- **Herbs and Spices**: Stock up on dried herbs (e.g., oregano, thyme, basil) and bold spices (e.g., cumin, turmeric, cayenne). These add layers of flavor without any salt. Fresh herbs, such as parsley, cilantro, and chives, also make excellent additions.
- **Low-Sodium Canned Goods**: Many brands offer low-sodium or no-salt-added canned goods like beans, tomatoes, and vegetables. If these aren't available, rinse regular canned items underwater to reduce the sodium content.
- **Citrus Fruits**: Lemons, limes, and oranges are flavor powerhouses. Their zest and juice can brighten up soups, salads, roasted meats, and more, making them an excellent salt replacement.
- **Vinegar**: Add tang and complexity to meals with vinegar like apple cider, balsamic, or red wine. They're excellent for marinades, dressings, and even drizzled-over vegetables.
- **Unsalted Nuts and Seeds**: Nuts and seeds make great snacks or salad toppers. Look for unsalted versions to keep sodium levels low.

- ***Garlic and Onion***: Fresh or powdered (without added salt), garlic and onion form the base of many flavorful dishes. Roasting them brings out their natural sweetness and depth.
- ***Healthy Fats***: Olive oil, avocado oil, or sesame oil add richness to meals while helping you absorb nutrients from other ingredients. These fats also balance flavors, making dishes feel more satisfying.

These are just a few examples of healthy, low-sodium ingredients that can be used in place of salt. Experiment with different herbs, spices, and other flavor-boosting ingredients to find combinations that suit your taste preferences. And don't forget to read nutrition labels and choose low-sodium options whenever possible.

Tips for Enhancing Flavor Without Salt

Cooking without salt doesn't mean sacrificing flavor. By using the right techniques and additions, you can build bold, appetizing dishes that taste far from bland.

1. ***Layer Flavors Gradually***: Think of cooking as building a masterpiece. Start with bold base flavors—like garlic, onion, or leeks—and layer additional flavors slowly. Add spices, herbs, or citrus throughout the cooking process to deepen the profile of your meal.

2. *Use High-Impact Ingredients*: Certain ingredients pack a punch and can transform your dish. For example, a splash of balsamic vinegar, a sprinkle of smoked paprika, or a dollop of mustard can add complexity without a hint of salt.
3. *Try Smoked or Roasted Items*: Roasting or grilling vegetables and proteins creates caramelized, smoky flavors that add depth. For example, roasted sweet potatoes or grilled zucchini can make a meal feel hearty and flavorful, all without a grain of salt.
4. *Experiment with Aromatics*: Sauté aromatics like ginger, shallots, garlic, or curry leaves before cooking your main ingredients. This infuses the dish with rich scents and tastes without needing added sodium.
5. *Rely on Acidity*: Acidic ingredients—such as vinegar, citrus juice, or even unsweetened yogurt—add brightness and can mimic some of the flavor-enhancing qualities of salt. Use them to finish recipes like salads, soups, or stir-fries.
6. *Boost Umami Flavor*: Umami, that savory "fifth taste," can add depth without salt. Ingredients like mushrooms, unsalted tomato paste, nutritional yeast, or fermented products like miso (low-sodium versions) bring that rich, satisfying quality to your dishes.
7. *Finish with Fresh Herbs*: Adding fresh herbs after cooking instantly livens up your dish. Basil, mint, parsley, or dill work beautifully as garnishes.

8. *Use Infused Oils*: Drizzle a small amount of infused oil, like garlic or chili oil, over dishes before serving for a gourmet finishing touch. A little goes a long way to add flavor.
9. *Focus on Textures*: Play with crunchy, creamy, or chewy textures to make meals more interesting. Adding a handful of toasted, unsalted nuts or a dollop of Greek yogurt (unsalted) can elevate how satisfying a dish feels.
10. *Taste as You Go*: Cooking low-sodium meals often means thinking creatively. Taste frequently during the process to ensure the flavors are balanced, and adjust with spices, acidity, or herbs as needed.

Cooking low-sodium meals at home is about getting creative and making the most of nature's flavors. With the right ingredients and techniques, you can enjoy dishes that are both healthy and delicious.

For seniors, this focus on low sodium can make a huge difference in managing blood pressure, heart health, and kidney health, all while keeping your taste buds happy. Whether it's a hearty soup, a fresh salad, or a roasted veggie side dish, the possibilities are endless when you cook with care and flavor in mind.

Dining Out Without Worry

Eating out can be a treat, but for those managing sodium intake, it can feel like navigating a tricky maze. With hidden salts lurking in menu items, it's easy to feel overwhelmed. But dining out and sticking to a low-sodium diet doesn't have to be at odds. By knowing what to look for and how to communicate your needs, you can enjoy meals outside of your home without worry.

1. **Study the Menu Ahead of Time**

    Before heading out, look up the restaurant's menu online. Many places now provide nutritional information, including sodium content. This can help you narrow down low-sodium choices in advance, saving you time and stress at the table.

2. **Focus on Simple, Fresh Foods**

    Menu items that are fresh, grilled, broiled, or steamed tend to have less sodium than fried or heavily sauced dishes. Consider dishes like grilled fish, steamed vegetables, or a fresh salad with dressing on the side.

3. **Avoid Pre-Made Sauces and Seasonings**

   Many sauces, marinades, and spice blends are loaded with sodium. Opt for grilled meats or fish without added sauces, or ask for them on the side so you can control how much you use.

4. **Watch Out for Soups and Appetizers**

   Soups, even ones that sound healthy like vegetable or chicken noodles, are often high in sodium due to stock and seasonings. Similarly, appetizers like chips, fries, or mozzarella sticks are heavily salted. Skip these in favor of a side salad or plain fruit.

5. **Swap Sides**

   Avoid traditional sides like fries, mashed potatoes (often loaded with salted butter), or rice pilaf. Instead, ask for steamed or sautéed vegetables, a baked potato (hold the salted toppings), or a fresh fruit cup.

6. **DIY Dressing and Condiments**

   Stick to oil and vinegar for salads instead of pre-made dressings, which frequently contain hidden sodium. For sandwiches or burgers, skip salty condiments like ketchup, pickles, or barbecue sauce unless there's a low-sodium alternative.

7. **Stay Hydrated**

    Sodium can leave you feeling thirsty and bloated. To help counteract this, drink plenty of water with your meal instead of salty beverages like sodas or alcoholic cocktails, both of which can make matters worse.

Overall, the key to reducing sodium in your restaurant meals is to be mindful and ask questions. Don't be afraid to request modifications or substitutions and always read menus carefully. By making smart choices and being aware of hidden sources of sodium, you can still enjoy dining out while maintaining a healthy diet.

How to Communicate Your Needs

One of the most important parts of dining out on a low-sodium diet is speaking up. Restaurant staff are there to help, but communication is key. Here's how to make your dietary needs clear without feeling uncomfortable.

1. **Be Polite But Direct**

    You don't have to explain every detail of your diet, but being upfront is important. Say something like, "I'm watching my sodium intake for health reasons. Can you help me make a good choice from the menu?" A smile and kindness go a long way in getting good service.

2. **Ask Questions**

   Don't hesitate to ask about how a dish is prepared. Questions like, "What seasonings are used?" or "Are these vegetables cooked with butter or salt?" can help you make an informed choice. If an item comes with a sauce or gravy, ask if it can be served on the side or skipped altogether.

3. **Request Modifications**

   Restaurants are often happy to adjust meals to suit dietary restrictions. You can ask for less salt to be used during preparation or have items like grilled chicken or vegetables served plain. Many chefs are used to making accommodations and will appreciate specific requests.

4. **Use Keywords**

   Phrases like "no added salt," "sauce on the side," and "steamed instead of sautéed" are simple ways to communicate exactly what you need.

5. **Speak to the Manager or Chef if Necessary**

   If your server isn't sure about sodium content or preparation methods, politely ask to speak with the chef or manager. They are often the most knowledgeable about what's going into the food and how it can be adjusted.

6. **Use Apps or Tools**

   Some apps provide sodium ratings for popular chain restaurant dishes. These can help you make a quick choice if you're unsure how to proceed.

7. **Celebrate the Wins**

   If the restaurant is able to accommodate your requests, make sure to thank the staff and leave positive feedback. Not only does it make the experience better for everyone, but it encourages more restaurants to provide flexibility for individuals with dietary requirements.

With a little preparation and communication, dining out on a low-sodium diet can be just as enjoyable as eating at home. Keep in mind that you're in control of what you order, and most restaurants are willing to work with you to meet your needs.

Over time, these strategies will become second nature, making it easier than ever to balance managing your sodium intake with enjoying great meals and dining experiences wherever you go.

7-Day Low-Sodium Meal Plan for Seniors

Eating a low-sodium diet doesn't mean giving up delicious, satisfying meals! This 7-day meal plan for seniors offers a balanced selection of breakfast, lunch, dinner, and snacks, all designed to keep sodium levels in check while maintaining taste and variety. Each day features wholesome ingredients, thoughtful preparation, and practical tips to make low-sodium eating enjoyable and easy.

Day 1

Breakfast: Oatmeal with Fresh Berries and Almonds

Snack: Sliced apple with unsalted peanut butter.

Lunch: Grilled Chicken Salad

Snack: Unsalted rice cakes with mashed avocado and a squeeze of fresh lime.

Dinner: Baked Salmon with Steamed Broccoli and Brown Rice

Day 2

Breakfast: Greek Yogurt Parfait

Snack: A handful of unsalted walnuts with a small tangerine.

Lunch: Quinoa and Vegetable Stir-Fry

Snack: Baby carrots and celery sticks with hummus (low-sodium version).

Dinner: Herb-Roasted Chicken Thighs with Mashed Sweet Potatoes and Green Beans

Day 3

Breakfast: Spinach and Mushroom Omelette

Snack: Fresh pear slices with unsalted almonds.

Lunch: Turkey Wrap

Snack: Cucumber slices with a light sprinkle of nutritional yeast for extra flavor.

Dinner: Lemon-garlic Cod with Roasted Vegetables

Day 4

Breakfast: Smoothie Bowl

Snack: Unsalted trail mix with dried cranberries, pumpkin seeds, and cashews.

Lunch: Lentil Soup with Side Salad

Snack: A hard-boiled egg with a dash of black pepper and paprika.

Dinner: Grilled Pork Tenderloin with Cauliflower Mash and Roasted Brussels Sprouts

Day 5

Breakfast: Whole-grain English Muffin with Avocado and Tomato

Snack: Fresh orange wedges with unsalted sunflower seeds.

Lunch: Stuffed Bell Peppers

Snack: Low-sodium cottage cheese with sliced cucumber and ground black pepper.

Dinner: Turkey Meatballs with Whole-Wheat Spaghetti

Day 6

Breakfast: Banana Pancakes

Snack: Celery sticks with unsalted almond butter.

Lunch: Chicken and Veggie Kabobs

Snack: Fresh pineapple chunks with unsalted cashews.

Dinner: Vegetable Stir-Fry with Tofu

Day 7

Breakfast: Veggie Breakfast Hash

Snack: A rice cake topped with hummus and sliced cherry tomatoes.

Lunch: Baked Salmon Salad

Snack: A cup of unsweetened Greek yogurt with a sprinkle of cinnamon and chopped pecans.

Dinner: Slow-Cooked Beef Stew

Final Tips for Success

- Use herbs, spices, and acidity (lemon, vinegar) to boost flavor without salt.
- Plan meals and snacks ahead to reduce temptation and stay on track.
- Opt for fresh or frozen produce and whole foods to avoid hidden sodium.
- Taste as you go when cooking to ensure meals are flavorful and well-balanced.

With this 7-day plan, you can mix and match meals or repeat your favorites. This will help keep your sodium intake low while still enjoying delicious, nutritious food every day!

Quick and Easy Low-Sodium Recipes

Eating a low-sodium diet doesn't have to be boring or difficult. Here's a collection of 20 flavorful and nutritious dishes, including 5 heart-healthy soups and salads, 10 satisfying main dishes, and 5 sweet yet low-sodium desserts. These recipes are simple to prepare, packed with flavor, and perfect for seniors looking to make healthy choices without giving up on taste.

Lentil and Spinach Soup

Ingredients:

- 2 tablespoons olive oil
- 1 medium onion, chopped
- 3 cloves garlic, minced
- 1 cup dried lentils, rinsed and drained
- 4 cups low-sodium vegetable broth
- 1 can (14.5 ounces) diced tomatoes, undrained
- 1 teaspoon dried thyme
- Salt and pepper to taste (omit salt for a low-sodium option)
- 4 cups fresh spinach leaves, roughly chopped

Instructions:

1. In a large pot, heat olive oil over medium heat.
2. Add onions and garlic and cook until softened.
3. Stir in lentils and cook for about one minute.
4. Pour in vegetable broth and bring to a boil.
5. Reduce heat and let simmer for 20 minutes, stirring occasionally.
6. Add diced tomatoes and dried thyme to the pot.
7. Let simmer for an additional 10 minutes or until lentils are tender.
8. Season with salt and pepper (if desired).
9. Stir in spinach leaves and cook until wilted.
10. Serve hot and enjoy!

Creamy Avocado and Cucumber Salad

Ingredients:

- 2 medium cucumbers, peeled and diced
- 1 avocado, peeled and diced
- 1 tablespoon fresh dill, chopped
- 1 tablespoon fresh chives, chopped
- 3 tablespoons plain Greek yogurt
- Salt and pepper to taste (omit salt for a low-sodium option)

Instructions:

1. In a large bowl, combine diced cucumbers and avocado.
2. Add in chopped dill and chives.
3. Stir in Greek yogurt until well combined.
4. Season with salt and pepper (if desired).
5. Serve as a side salad or enjoy on its own!

Tomato Basil Soup

Ingredients:

- 4 cups low-sodium canned diced tomatoes
- 2 cups low-sodium vegetable broth
- 1 onion, chopped
- 2 cloves garlic, minced
- 1/4 cup fresh basil, chopped (plus extra for garnish)

Instructions:

1. In a large pot, heat olive oil over medium heat.
2. Add onions and garlic and cook until softened.
3. Pour in diced tomatoes and vegetable broth.
4. Bring to a boil, then reduce heat and let simmer for 20 minutes.
5. Using an immersion blender, puree the soup until smooth.
6. Stir in chopped basil and let simmer for an additional 10 minutes.
7. Serve hot with extra chopped basil as garnish.

Rainbow Quinoa Salad

Ingredients:

- 1 cup cooked quinoa
- 1 cup chopped bell peppers (red, yellow, and green)
- 1/2 cup shredded carrots
- 1/4 cup chopped parsley
- 2 tbsp olive oil
- 1 tbsp apple cider vinegar

Instructions:

1. In a large bowl, combine cooked quinoa and chopped bell peppers.
2. Stir in shredded carrots and parsley.
3. In a small bowl, whisk together olive oil and apple cider vinegar.
4. Pour dressing over salad and toss to combine.
5. Serve as a side dish or add protein (such as grilled chicken or tofu) for a complete meal.

Vegetable Barley Soup

Ingredients:

- 1/2 cup pearl barley
- 6 cups low-sodium vegetable broth
- 1 cup chopped carrots
- 1 cup celery slices
- 1 cup diced tomatoes (no salt added)
- 1 tsp thyme

Instructions:

1. In a large pot, combine pearl barley and vegetable broth.
2. Bring to a boil, then reduce heat and let simmer for 30 minutes.
3. Add chopped carrots, celery slices, diced tomatoes, and thyme to the pot.
4. Let simmer for an additional 20 minutes until vegetables are tender.
5. Serve hot as a hearty and healthy soup option. You can also add in other vegetables such as broccoli or cauliflower for added nutrients and flavor.

Lemon Herb Chicken

Ingredients:

- 4 boneless, skinless chicken breasts
- 2 cloves garlic, minced
- 1 lemon, juiced and zested
- 2 tbsp olive oil
- 1 tsp dried rosemary
- Salt and pepper to taste

Instructions:

1. In a small bowl, whisk together minced garlic, lemon juice and zest, olive oil, dried rosemary, salt and pepper.
2. Place chicken breasts in a resealable plastic bag or shallow dish.
3. Pour marinade over chicken and let marinate for at least an hour (or up to overnight) in the fridge.
4. Preheat the grill or grill pan to medium-high heat.
5. Remove chicken from marinade and discard excess marinade.
6. Grill chicken for 6-7 minutes on each side, until cooked through and no longer pink in the middle.

7. Serve hot with your choice of sides, such as roasted vegetables or a salad.
8. For added flavor, you can also sprinkle some additional dried rosemary on top of the chicken before grilling.

Grilled Salmon with Dill Sauce

Ingredients:

- 4 salmon fillets
- 1/4 cup plain Greek yogurt
- 1 tbsp Dijon mustard
- 1 tsp dried dill
- Salt and pepper to taste

Instructions:

1. Preheat the grill or grill pan to medium-high heat.
2. In a small bowl, mix together Greek yogurt, Dijon mustard, dried dill, salt and pepper.
3. Place salmon fillets on the preheated grill and cook for about 5 minutes on each side, until cooked through and flaky.
4. Serve hot with a dollop of the dill sauce on top of each fillet.
5. For added flavor, you can also add some fresh lemon slices on top of the salmon before grilling.

Stuffed Bell Peppers

Ingredients:

- 4 bell peppers (any color)
- 1 lb ground beef or turkey
- 1 cup cooked rice
- 1 can diced tomatoes, drained
- 1/2 onion, diced
- 2 cloves garlic, minced
- 1 tsp dried oregano
- Salt and pepper to taste

Instructions:

1. Preheat oven to 375°F.
2. Cut the tops off of each bell pepper and remove seeds and membranes from inside.
3. In a skillet, cook ground beef or turkey over medium heat until browned. Drain excess fat.
4. Add in diced onions, minced garlic, dried oregano, salt and pepper to skillet. Cook for another 2-3 minutes.
5. Stir in cooked rice and drained diced tomatoes into the skillet with the meat mixture.
6. Fill each bell pepper with the meat and rice mixture.

7. Place filled peppers in a baking dish and bake for 25-30 minutes until peppers are soft and the filling is heated through.
8. Serve hot as is, or top with shredded cheese before serving for an extra gooey treat.

Zucchini Noodles with Garlic Shrimp

Ingredients:

- 2 medium zucchini
- 1 lb shrimp, peeled and deveined
- 4 cloves garlic, minced
- 1/4 cup olive oil
- Salt and pepper to taste

Instructions:

1. Using a spiralizer or vegetable peeler, create long thin strips of zucchini noodles.
2. Heat up olive oil in a large skillet over medium heat.
3. Add in minced garlic and cook for about one minute until fragrant.
4. Add shrimp to the skillet and cook until pink and cooked through (about 5 minutes).
5. Stir in zucchini noodles and cook for another 2 minutes until noodles are slightly softened.
6. Season with salt and pepper to taste.
7. Serve hot as is, or top with grated parmesan cheese for an extra savory touch.

Vegetarian Stir-Fry

Ingredients:

- 1 cup cooked rice
- 2 bell peppers, sliced
- 1 onion, sliced
- 1 cup broccoli florets
- 1 cup carrots, sliced
- 1 cup mushrooms, sliced
- 1/4 cup soy sauce
- 2 tbsp sesame oil

Instructions:

1. In a large skillet or wok, heat up sesame oil over medium-high heat.
2. Add bell peppers, onions, broccoli, carrots, and mushrooms to the skillet and cook for about 5 minutes until vegetables are slightly softened.
3. Stir in cooked rice and soy sauce into the vegetable mixture.
4. Cook for another 2-3 minutes until rice is heated through and coated in soy sauce.
5. Serve hot as a vegetarian meal or top with grilled chicken or tofu for added protein.
6. For an extra kick of flavor, sprinkle some red pepper flakes on top before serving.

Turkey and Avocado Wrap

Ingredients:

- 4 large whole wheat tortillas
- 1 lb cooked turkey, sliced
- 2 avocados, sliced
- 1 tomato, diced
- 1/4 cup shredded cheddar cheese
- Salt and pepper to taste

Instructions:

1. Lay out tortillas on a flat surface.
2. In the center of each tortilla, layer slices of turkey, avocado, tomato, and shredded cheese.
3. Season with salt and pepper to taste.
4. Roll up the tortillas tightly into wraps.
5. Heat up a skillet or pan over medium heat.
6. Place wraps seam side down on the skillet and cook for 2-3 minutes until the tortilla is lightly browned.
7. Flip the wraps over and cook for another 2-3 minutes on the other side.
8. Serve hot as a healthy and satisfying lunch option.

Rosemary Pork Chops

Ingredients:

- 4 pork chops
- 2 tbsp olive oil
- 1 tsp dried rosemary
- Salt and pepper to taste

Instructions:

1. Preheat oven to 375°F.
2. Season pork chops with salt, pepper, and dried rosemary on both sides.
3. Heat up olive oil in a large skillet over medium-high heat.
4. Once the oil is hot, add in pork chops and cook for about 5 minutes on each side until browned.
5. Transfer pork chops to a baking dish and bake in a preheated oven for 15-20 minutes or until cooked through.
6. Serve hot with your choice of side dishes, such as roasted vegetables or mashed potatoes.

Vegetable and Chickpea Curry

Ingredients:

- 1 can chickpeas, drained and rinsed
- 1 can diced tomatoes (low-sodium)
- 1/2 cup coconut milk
- 2 cups mixed vegetables (such as cauliflower, carrots, bell peppers, and peas)
- 2 tbsp curry powder
- Salt to taste
- Cooked brown rice for serving

Instructions:

1. In a large pot or saucepan, combine chickpeas, diced tomatoes, coconut milk, mixed vegetables, curry powder.
2. Bring mixture to a simmer over medium heat.
3. Reduce heat to low and let it simmer for about 10 minutes until the vegetables are cooked and the flavors have melded together.
4. Season with salt to taste.
5. Serve over a bed of cooked brown rice for a complete meal.

Baked Cod with Lemon and Garlic

Ingredients:

- 4 cod fillets
- 2 tbsp olive oil
- Juice of 1 lemon
- 4 cloves garlic, minced
- Salt and pepper to taste

Instructions:

1. Preheat oven to 375°F.
2. Place cod fillets in a baking dish and drizzle olive oil over them.
3. Squeeze lemon juice over the fish and sprinkle minced garlic on top.
4. Season with salt and pepper to taste.
5. Bake in preheated oven for about 15 minutes or until the fish flakes easily with a fork.
6. Serve hot as a light and flavorful dinner option.

Beef and Vegetable Skewers

Ingredients:

- 1 lb beef sirloin, cut into cubes
- 2 bell peppers, cut into chunks
- 1 red onion, cut into chunks
- 8 cherry tomatoes
- Salt and pepper to taste

Instructions:

1. Preheat the grill or grill pan to medium-high heat.
2. Assemble skewers by alternating beef cubes with bell pepper, onion, and tomato.
3. Season with salt and pepper on all sides of the skewers.
4. Grill for about 10 minutes, turning occasionally, until beef is cooked to desired doneness and vegetables are slightly charred.
5. Serve hot as a tasty and nutritious meal.

Fresh Berry Yogurt Parfait

Ingredients:

- 1 cup unsweetened Greek yogurt
- 1/2 cup fresh strawberries, sliced
- 1/2 cup fresh blueberries
- 1/4 cup unsalted granola

Instructions:

1. In a small parfait glass or bowl, layer the Greek yogurt with sliced strawberries and blueberries.
2. Top with a sprinkle of unsalted granola for added crunch.
3. Repeat layers until ingredients are used up.
4. Serve immediately as a light and healthy dessert option.

Baked Apples with Cinnamon

Ingredients:

- 4 apples
- 1/2 cup oats
- 1/4 cup raisins
- Cinnamon to taste

Instructions:

1. Preheat oven to 350°F.
2. Slice off the top of each apple and use a spoon or melon baller to remove the core, making sure not to pierce through the bottom.
3. In a small bowl, mix together oats and raisins with a sprinkle of cinnamon.
4. Stuff each apple with the oat mixture, pressing down lightly to compact it inside.
5. Place stuffed apples in a baking dish and bake for about 20 minutes, until soft and slightly golden on top.
6. Serve warm as a comforting and healthy dessert option.

Chia Seed Pudding

Ingredients:

- 1/4 cup chia seeds
- 1 cup unsweetened almond milk
- Splash of vanilla extract
- Fresh fruit for topping (optional)

Instructions:

1. In a bowl or jar, mix together chia seeds, almond milk, and vanilla extract.
2. Cover and refrigerate for at least 4 hours or overnight.
3. When ready to serve, top with fresh fruit if desired.
4. Enjoy as a healthy and filling breakfast or snack option.

Banana Ice Cream

Ingredients:

- 2 ripe bananas, sliced and frozen
- Optional: cocoa powder for sprinkling

Instructions:

1. In a blender or food processor, add frozen banana slices.
2. Blend until smooth and creamy, scraping down the sides as needed.
3. Serve immediately as a healthy and simple dessert option.
4. For added flavor, sprinkle some cocoa powder on top before serving.

Dark Chocolate-Dipped Strawberries

Ingredients:

- 1 cup unsweetened dark chocolate chips
- Fresh strawberries

Instructions:

1. In a microwave-safe bowl, microwave the chocolate chips in 30-second intervals, stirring in between until completely melted.
2. Dip fresh strawberries into the melted chocolate and place on parchment paper.
3. Place in the fridge to set for about 10 minutes before serving.
4. Enjoy as a decadent and healthy treat option.

This low-sodium recipe is designed to keep meals flavorful, varied, and satisfying. With these soups, salads, main dishes, and desserts in your arsenal, eating a low-sodium diet becomes an exciting adventure full of options.

Tracking Your Sodium Intake

Managing sodium intake is an essential step for seniors aiming to maintain good health and prevent heart-related issues. Tracking your sodium consumption can help you stay on course with your dietary goals, and with the right tools and strategies, it doesn't have to feel overwhelming. This guide will walk you through practical ways to monitor and manage sodium intake, deal with cravings, and know when to seek professional help.

Journals, Apps, and Tools for Seniors

Food Journals

Writing down everything you eat in a food journal is a simple and effective way to monitor sodium levels. Use a notebook or printed food diary templates to record meals, snacks, beverages, and sodium content.

- Track your daily sodium intake in milligrams.
- Write down any high-sodium foods or situations where you might slip up, so you can plan better next time.

- Reflect on your journal weekly to identify patterns and make adjustments.

Apps for Tracking

There are many apps designed to help track sodium intake. Choose one that's easy to use and senior-friendly. Some popular options include:

- *MyFitnessPal*: Tracks overall nutrition, including sodium.
- *Sodium Tracker*: Designed specifically to monitor sodium intake per meal.
- *Lose It!*: Helps you set custom nutrition goals.

Most apps allow you to scan barcodes or search for foods to get a quick sodium count. Many also feature reminders to log your meals and snacks.

Helpful Tools

- *Digital Food Scales*: These are essential tools for accurately measuring portion sizes, which can help you better manage your sodium intake. By weighing ingredients, you can ensure you're staying within your dietary goals and tracking sodium levels more precisely.
- *Salt-Free Herb Blends*: Stock up on jarred spice mixes that contain a variety of herbs and spices to replace salt in your recipes. These blends are a great

way to add depth and flavor to your meals while keeping them healthy and sodium-free. Try experimenting with different combinations to find your favorites.

- ***Sodium-Free Recipe Books***: These cookbooks are packed with ideas and inspiration for creating delicious, flavorful meals without relying on added salt. They often include tips for substituting salt, using fresh ingredients, and enhancing natural flavors, making them a valuable resource in your kitchen.

Staying Consistent

Building habits takes time, so it's important to stay consistent with your sodium-tracking routine. Here are a few tips to make it easier:

- ***Set Daily Goals***: Start by understanding your recommended daily sodium limit, which is typically 2,300 mg or less, unless your doctor advises otherwise. Break this down into smaller targets for each meal to help you stay on track throughout the day. Keeping an eye on your intake can make a big difference in managing your health.
- ***Create a Routine***: Make logging your meals a consistent habit by choosing a time that fits seamlessly into your schedule, such as after meals, during your lunch break, or while relaxing in the evening. Using a

food diary or an app can make tracking easier and more accurate.
- **Batch Cook Meals**: Take some time each week to prepare low-sodium meals in advance. Cooking in batches not only makes healthy eating more convenient but also helps you avoid the temptation of high-sodium snacks or takeout on busy days. Store meals in portion-sized containers for quick access throughout the week.

Reward yourself for sticking to your plan! Treating yourself to a non-food-related reward, like a new book or a relaxing day out, can motivate you to maintain consistency.

Dealing with Cravings and Setbacks

Understanding Cravings

Salt cravings often stem from habits or emotional triggers. These cravings may arise if you've consumed salty foods for a long time or when you feel stressed or bored.

How to Handle Setbacks

- **Learn from Them**: If you eat something high in sodium, take a moment to reflect on why it happened. Was it due to convenience, stress, or being unprepared? Understanding the reason can help you make better choices in the future. Use it as a learning opportunity rather than a reason to feel discouraged or give up on your goals.

- ***Stay Positive***: One high-sodium meal won't derail your progress or undo all your hard work. What matters is how you move forward. Focus on getting back on track with your next meal by choosing low-sodium, nutrient-dense options. Remember, progress is about consistency, not perfection, so don't beat yourself up over small mistakes.

- ***Keep Low-Sodium Snacks Available***: Having something satisfying and healthy on hand, like unsalted nuts, fresh fruit, or raw veggies, can help curb salty cravings before they take over. Planning ahead ensures you're prepared when hunger strikes, making it easier to avoid reaching for high-sodium options. Small steps like these can make a big difference in maintaining your goals.

Tips for Managing Salt Cravings

Salt cravings don't mean you have to sacrifice flavor. Here are ways to combat those cravings while sticking to your low-sodium goals:

1. ***Use Fresh Herbs and Spices***: Fresh herbs like basil, cilantro, and rosemary, and spices such as paprika and pepper, can naturally enhance the flavor of your dishes without adding unhealthy ingredients. They not only

provide aromatic depth but also bring vibrant, distinct tastes to any meal. Try experimenting with combinations to suit your cuisine!

2. *Add Acidity*: Brighten up flavors by incorporating a splash of lemon juice, lime juice, or vinegar. Acidity helps balance tastes and can elevate the overall flavor profile of your dish, making it taste fresher and more vibrant. It's a simple way to replace salt while enhancing zest.

3. *Try Aromatic Additions*: Ingredients like garlic, onion, ginger, and scallions can infuse your meals with richness and complexity. Sauté them for a delicious base or add them fresh for a bold punch of flavor—these staples are essential for creating layered and satisfying dishes.

4. *Experiment with Umami*: Add a savory, satisfying depth to your meals with umami-rich ingredients such as mushrooms, sun-dried tomatoes, or nutritional yeast. These elements bring a hearty, almost meaty taste that can make vegetarian or plant-based dishes taste indulgent and full of flavor.

Often, cravings fade after 10–15 minutes. During this time, redirect your attention to an activity you enjoy, like reading or going for a walk.

Staying Motivated

Tracking sodium and changing habits is a big lifestyle shift. Staying motivated is crucial to your long-term success.

- *Focus on Small Wins*: Celebrate every day you meet your sodium goal or even every low-sodium meal you enjoy. It's the small, consistent steps that lead to big changes over time. Treat every success as a reason to keep going, whether it's picking a healthier snack or cooking a homemade, low-sodium dish.
- *Find a Support System*: Share your goals with family or friends. Having someone to cheer you on can make a huge difference, and they might even decide to join you in adopting healthier eating habits. You can cook together, swap recipes, or simply encourage one another to stay on track when things get tough.
- *Visualize Your Outcome*: Remind yourself of the benefits you're working toward, like better blood pressure, improved heart health, and more energy every day. Picture how it will feel to wake up with more vitality or to know you're doing something great for your long-term health. Keeping these benefits in mind can keep you motivated when making changes feels challenging.

Writing down your motivation and rereading it regularly can serve as a powerful reminder to keep going, even when it feels challenging.

When to Consult a Doctor or Dietitian

Managing sodium intake can be challenging, and consulting a healthcare professional can provide the guidance and reassurance you need to stay on track. Below, we'll expand on the key scenarios when reaching out to a doctor or dietitian is essential:

Medical Conditions

Certain health conditions make it especially important to control sodium levels. A doctor or dietitian can help by offering specific sodium limits and tailored advice based on your medical history and overall health.

1. **High Blood Pressure**

    Reduced sodium intake directly impacts blood pressure levels. A doctor can assess your current blood pressure and recommend an optimal sodium cap—often lower than the standard 2,300 mg per day. They may also suggest monitoring devices or medications to complement dietary changes. A dietitian can guide you toward sodium-friendly meals while ensuring you get adequate nutrition.

2. **Kidney Disease**

   When kidneys do not function properly, the body struggles to eliminate excess sodium, which can lead to fluid retention. Medical professionals can design a low-sodium diet that also limits other high-risk nutrients, like potassium and phosphorus. This ensures your kidney health is managed holistically.

3. **Congestive Heart Failure (CHF)**

   Too much sodium can worsen heart failure symptoms by causing fluid buildup. A medical professional can teach you how to balance sodium intake alongside monitoring fluids. They may also help you understand food labels better, so you can easily identify and avoid high-sodium products.

For other chronic conditions, such as diabetes or liver diseases, specialized sodium guidance can help slow disease progression and improve quality of life. Scheduling regular consultations allows your care team to adapt recommendations as your condition changes.

Plateaus or Challenges

No matter how dedicated you are to reducing sodium intake, there might be times when progress stalls or challenges feel overwhelming. This is normal, and professional guidance can help you overcome these hurdles.

1. **Plateaus**

    If your progress levels off—for instance, your blood pressure stops improving despite maintaining a low-sodium diet—a dietitian can evaluate your food choices for hidden sodium sources. They can also experiment with small adjustments, like incorporating new low-sodium staples or revising portion sizes, to optimize your results.

2. **Challenges in Adherence**

    Struggling to stick to your plan? A professional can help you identify the root cause. For example, you may unknowingly be choosing foods with high "hidden sodium," such as bread or restaurant dishes. A dietitian can suggest alternatives and offer practical tips, like meal-prepping low-sodium options or carrying homemade snacks on the go.

3. **Motivational Setbacks**

    Frustration or cravings may cause you to revert to old habits. A dietitian can introduce "mindful eating" practices to help you manage emotions tied to food and suggest flavorful substitutes for your favorite salty snacks. Remember, there's no one-size-fits-all solution—professionals tailor their approach to what works best for you.

Custom Plans

One of the most valuable resources a dietitian can provide is a personalized meal plan designed specifically for your health goals, lifestyle, and food preferences.

1. **Meeting Health Goals**

    Whether you aim to control high blood pressure, reduce fluid retention, or prevent future health complications, a dietitian can create a plan that balances sodium reduction with adequate protein, fiber, and other nutrients your body needs. They may also account for other dietary restrictions, such as managing diabetes or food allergies.

2. **Tailored to Your Preferences**

    A dietitian takes the time to understand your likes and dislikes. For example, if you enjoy hearty soups or baked goods, they can suggest low-sodium broth alternatives or baking tips that result in satisfying, low-sodium versions of your favorite dishes. This personalization makes sticking to the plan easier and more enjoyable.

3. **Culturally Inclusive Options**

   Eating habits are culturally influenced, and food traditions are important to preserve. A dietitian understands this and can work within your cultural preferences, ensuring you don't feel restricted from enjoying your heritage's cuisine. For example, they may offer ideas for seasoning blends that replicate traditional flavors without added salt.

Custom plans come with built-in flexibility so you can adjust to life's unpredictability, like travel or social events. Plus, they empower you to become more confident in making low-sodium choices on your own.

Managing sodium isn't just about reading labels or limiting certain foods—it's about adopting a lifestyle that balances health and joy. A professional's expertise provides you with tools, knowledge, and encouragement to make sustainable changes. By consulting your doctor or dietitian when needed, you're prioritizing both your present well-being and your long-term health goals.

Recognizing When You Need Help

Managing sodium intake can be challenging, and there may be times when you feel it's difficult to stay on track. Recognizing these moments and seeking support can make a significant difference. Here's a closer look at some common scenarios and how to handle them:

1. **Feeling Overwhelmed or Burnt Out**

   If keeping track of sodium intake feels like too much work or is draining your energy, it's important to recognize this as a sign to adjust your approach.

   - *Ask for Family Support*: You don't have to do this alone. Ask a family member, friend, or caregiver to help you with meal prep, grocery shopping, or tracking your daily sodium intake. Even having someone assist you in reading food labels or planning your meals can make things easier and help you feel supported.
   - *Simplify Your Tracking System*: Instead of trying to track every single bite, focus on key meals or snacks that are typically higher in sodium. You can also use color-coded charts (green for low-sodium choices, and red for high-sodium) as quick visual aids. Additionally, consider digital apps that automate most of the tracking for you so that you don't need to write everything down manually.
   - *Take Small Steps*: If the adjustments feel overwhelming, start small. For example, swap out just one high-sodium item per week or gradually reduce your salt use during cooking. Small, manageable changes can build

confidence over time without feeling like a burden.

Feeling burnt out is normal when you're making lifestyle changes. By lightening the load and bringing loved ones into the process, you'll find it easier to stay the course.

2. **Experiencing Regular Slip-Ups**

If you're finding that high-sodium foods keep sneaking back into your diet, it's a sign that some routines or habits might need to be revisited.

- *Reflect on Your Patterns*: Look for the root causes of the slip-ups. Are you eating out more frequently than planned? Are you reaching for convenient packaged foods during busy days? Once you identify the issue, you can implement specific strategies to address it. For example, batch-cooking low-sodium meals or keeping pre-made snacks at hand could reduce the temptation of convenience foods.
- *Consult a Dietitian*: A dietitian can help you uncover hidden sources of sodium in your diet and suggest substitutions that fit your lifestyle. For instance, they might recommend low-sodium versions of your favorite snacks or teach you how to read food labels more

effectively. Dietitians are also great at problem-solving. Whether it's eating out, managing cravings, or finding better low-sodium flavors, they'll provide advice tailored to your needs.

- ***Practice Self-Compassion***: Slip-ups happen, and they don't mean you've failed. Instead of focusing on any missteps, use them as opportunities to learn and refine your dietary routine.

Regular slip-ups often highlight areas where a bit of creative planning or professional advice can make a big difference in staying consistent.

3. Noticing Health Changes

Physical symptoms like sudden weight fluctuations, swelling, or fatigue can be indicators that your sodium intake isn't aligning well with your body's needs. It's crucial to take these signs seriously and consult a doctor promptly.

- ***Weight Fluctuations and Fluid Retention***: These can often be linked to sodium intake causing excess water retention in the body. If you notice consistent bloating or shifts in your weight that are unrelated to other factors, a doctor can help pinpoint whether sodium or another issue is contributing to the changes. They may also check for underlying conditions, such as kidney or heart-related issues, that could require a stricter sodium limit.

- ***Swelling (Edema)***: Swelling in the legs, feet, or hands can be a sign of excess fluid retention due to high sodium consumption. A doctor might recommend reducing sodium further and could prescribe additional interventions to manage this.
- ***Fatigue or Lethargy***: If you feel overly tired or low-energy, it could be a sign of an electrolyte imbalance partly influenced by sodium consumption. Your doctor will evaluate whether your current sodium intake is appropriate and may suggest blood tests to rule out other medical concerns.

Consulting a professional when these health changes occur allows you to proactively address potential complications. It also ensures that your sodium guidelines are tailored to any new or evolving health needs.

Conclusion

Managing your sodium intake is more than adjusting your diet—it's actively taking charge of your health. By being mindful of the sodium in your meals, you're doing more than just reading labels or swapping salt for herbs. You're making choices that protect your heart, strengthen your body, and enhance your overall well-being. The benefits aren't distant or abstract; they're everyday improvements you can feel, like more energy, better control of your health, and peace of mind knowing you're supporting your body as it changes with age.

One of the biggest wins from managing sodium is the way it helps your heart. Too much sodium causes blood pressure to rise, which makes your heart work harder than it should. By cutting back, you're lightening this load and reducing your risk of heart disease, heart failure, or stroke. Each meal you plan or recipe you tweak is a step toward keeping your heart healthy and beating strong.

Your kidneys also benefit when you take sodium seriously. They work tirelessly to filter sodium and water from your body. But as you age, they can struggle to keep up, especially if you're consuming too much salt. By moderating your intake, you make it easier for your kidneys to do their job efficiently, minimizing risks like kidney disease or fluid retention.

Even your bones get a boost! High sodium can pull calcium out of your bones over time, increasing the risk of osteoporosis or fractures. When you stay on top of your sodium levels, you're helping to preserve bone strength, which means staying active and independent.

And those perks? They go far beyond numbers on a chart. You'll notice improvements in how you feel day-to-day. Less bloating, steadier energy, and fewer worries about how certain foods might affect you. You'll find it easier to keep up with hobbies, family gatherings, or even a stroll in the park. These are the moments that make all your efforts worthwhile.

The most rewarding part? Realizing you're the one in control. By learning what's in your food and recognizing hidden sodium sources, you're reclaiming your choices. It's not about giving up the tastes you love—it's about eating smart and making subtle changes that add up to big rewards. Think of it as investing in yourself every day.

You can cook flavorful, enjoyable meals without reaching for the salt shaker. You can ask questions at restaurants to ensure they prepare your dish to fit your needs. Every time you do, you're proving to yourself that you can shape your diet—and your future.

Remember, it's not about perfection. There's no harm in enjoying a meal out or indulging in a treat every now and then. What matters is the effort and consistency you bring to the bigger picture. Each choice you make, whether it's skipping salty snacks or seasoning with fresh herbs, shows your commitment to living well.

You've got the tools and know-how now, and that's no small thing. This is your health, your body, and your future to shape. Take what you've learned, keep experimenting in the kitchen, and lean on support when you need it. You're making a difference in your own life—and that deserves to be celebrated every step of the way.

FAQs

Why is sodium balance important, especially for seniors?

Sodium plays a crucial role in maintaining fluid balance, supporting muscle function, and transmitting nerve signals. However, as people age, kidney function may decline, making it harder to regulate sodium levels. This increases the risk of health issues like high blood pressure, heart problems, and bone density loss, making sodium management essential for seniors.

What is the recommended daily sodium intake for seniors?

Most seniors should aim for a daily sodium intake of 1,500 to 2,300 milligrams, depending on individual health needs. Seniors with conditions such as high blood pressure, heart disease, or kidney problems should stay closer to the lower limit (1,500 mg) to prevent complications.

What are the signs of consuming too much sodium?

Early signs include fluid retention (bloating or swelling in the hands and feet), increased thirst, and frequent urination. Over time, excessive sodium intake can lead to elevated blood pressure, persistent headaches, and even difficulty breathing. For seniors, this can worsen chronic conditions like heart or kidney disease.

What are some practical ways to reduce sodium in the diet?

To reduce sodium intake, opt for fresh fruits, vegetables, and whole foods while limiting processed and pre-packaged meals. Use herbs, spices, citrus juices, and vinegar to flavor food instead of salt. Reading nutrition labels, choosing "low-sodium" options, and preparing meals at home also help maintain sodium control.

What are common hidden sources of sodium in foods?

Sodium is often hidden in foods like bread, canned vegetables, soups, frozen meals, processed meats, and condiments like soy sauce, ketchup, and salad dressings. Always check nutrition labels for sodium content, even in products that don't taste salty.

Could Completely Removing Sodium from Your Diet Be Harmful?

Yes, sodium is an essential mineral for the body. Eliminating it entirely can cause issues like muscle cramps, confusion, and fatigue. Seniors should focus on reducing sodium to healthy levels rather than cutting it out completely, as balanced sodium intake is necessary for overall health.

How can seniors manage sodium intake when dining out or eating on the go?

Seniors can review menus ahead of time, opt for grilled, steamed, or fresh foods, and ask for sauces or dressings on the side. Avoid salty appetizers like soups or fries and request less salt in meal preparation. Be sure to communicate dietary needs politely and seek lower-sodium options whenever possible.

References and Helpful Links

Low sodium meal plans. (2023, January 4). EatingWell. https://www.eatingwell.com/category/4302/low-sodium-meal-plans/

Ms, H. P. (2023, May 11). 6 Little-Known Dangers of restricting sodium too much. Healthline. https://www.healthline.com/nutrition/6-dangers-of-sodium-restriction

Lindseyhurdadmin. (2024, February 5). 5 Ways for Seniors to Reduce sodium Consumption - The Alden Network. The Alden Network. https://www.alden.com/5-ways-for-seniors-to-reduce-sodium-consumption/

UCSF Health. (2024, May 21). Guidelines for a low sodium diet. ucsfhealth.org. https://www.ucsfhealth.org/education/guidelines-for-a-low-sodium-diet

A senior Guide to Low sodium diets. (2024, December 18). https://www.chestnutsquare.info/a-senior-guide-to-low-sodium-diets

Blood pressure UK. (n.d.). https://www.bloodpressureuk.org/your-blood-pressure/how-to-lower-your-blood-pressure/healthy-eating/salt-and-your-blood-pressure/

Loh, A. (2024, October 24). 30 Low-Sodium Dinners that support healthy aging. EatingWell.

https://www.eatingwell.com/gallery/7895976/healthy-aging-low-sodium-dinner-recipes/

www.ingramcontent.com/pod-product-compliance
Lightning Source LLC
LaVergne TN
LVHW012032060526
838201LV00061B/4572